TIGHT HIP FLEXOR

A Visual Manual On How To Completely Fix and Reduce Pains Like Magic

PERCY T. WILLIAMS

Copyright©2019

COPYRIGHT

No part of this publication may be reproduced, distributed, or transmitted in any form or by any means, including photocopying, recording, or other electronic or mechanical methods, or by any information storage and retrieval system without the prior written permission of the publisher, except in the case of very brief quotations embodied in critical reviews and certain other noncommercial uses per-mitted by copyright law

Percy T. Williams

TABLE OF CONTENT

CHAPTER ONE 4
    INTRODUCTION 4
CHAPTER TWO 7
    SYMPTOMS OF HIP FLEXOR 7
CHAPTER THREE 9
    CAUSES OF HIP FLEXOR 9
CHAPTER FOUR 11
    SIMPLE HIP FLEXOR STRETCHES TO PERFORM 11
CHAPTER FIVE 17
    HIP FLEXOR STRENGTHENING EXERCISES YOU SHOULD PERFORM 17
CHAPTER SIX 29
    RISKS ASSOCIATED WITH TIGHT HIP FLEXORS 29
CHAPTER SEVEN 31
    WHAT DIFFERENT TREATMENT APPROACH IS AVALIABLE? 31
CHAPTER EIGHT 35
    IMPORTANT TIPS TO PREVENT HIP FLEXOR 35
THE END 37

CHAPTER ONE

INTRODUCTION

People who sit for long periods of time are at a excessive threat of getting tight hip flexors. When hip flexors are tight, a man or woman may additionally experience pain in the decrease again and hips.

Tight hip flexors can also lead to injuries. Fortunately, there are numerous stretches and exercises that relax and improve the hip flexors. With improved strength and flexibility, a person is much less likely to have pain or injury.

Percy T. Williams

A person's hip flexors are the muscle groups that surround the ball and socket joints that join the legs to the top body.

These muscles are imperative to the motion of the lower body.

The hip flexors, which consist of 5 wonderful muscles, are frequently a left out muscle group.

It is not uncommon for even workout enthusiasts to leave out workout routines that toughen and stretch these muscles.

A man or woman need to maintain the hip flexors well-stretched and sturdy to assist avoid harm or forestall present injuries getting worse.

Tight Hip Flexor

CHAPTER TWO

SYMPTOMS OF HIP FLEXOR

Many humans who experience hip flexor strain will have these signs and symptoms as well:

a. Sudden, sharp ache in the hip or pelvis after trauma to the area

b. A cramping or clenching sensation in the muscle tissue of the top leg area

c. The top leg feeling smooth and sore

d. Loss of power in the front of the groin along with a tugging sensation

e. Muscle spasms in the hip or thighs

f. Inability to proceed kicking, jumping, or sprinting

g. Reduced mobility and pain when moving, such as limping

h. Discomfort and pain in the upper leg area, which feels constant

i. Swelling or bruising around the hip or thigh area

j. Tightness or stiffness after being stationary, such as after napping

CHAPTER THREE

CAUSES OF HIP FLEXOR

Dancing and jogging may put the hip flexor muscles under strain.

A person's hip flexors are engaged when they convey their knee up in the direction of their torso.

Hence, things to do such as dancing, martial arts, or strolling are the place hip flexors are put under the most strain.

Athletes who use the hip flexors in their game and education are more susceptible to hip flexor pressure or harm that can purpose the muscle groups to tear.

In sports activities medicine, it is notion that many hip flexor wounds are associated with hamstring strains

CHAPTER FOUR

SIMPLE HIP FLEXOR STRETCHES TO PERFORM

Several stretches will help enhance flexibility and make the hip flexors less prone to injury. Some workouts to stretch the hip flexors encompass the following:

Seated butterfly

The seated butterfly stretch stretches the hips, thighs, and decrease back. It is effortless to function and is accomplished from a seated position.

To carryout this stretch:

a. Sit up straight with engaged abs.
b. Push the bottoms of every foot together whilst pushing the knees out.
c. Pull heels toward the body and relax the knees, permitting them to flow toward the ground.
d. Hold for about 20 to 30 seconds, respiratory deeply.

Bridge pose

Bridge is a famous pose in yoga. It stretches many components of the legs, hips, and returned while lying down.

To carryout this stretch:

a. Lay flat on the ground with hands laid flat on both side.
b. Pull toes in the direction of the buttocks and maintain soles flat on the ground.
c. Engaging the core, elevate the buttocks into the air and shape a straight, angled line from the knees to the shoulders.

d. Hold for about 30 seconds, lower, and repeat.

Pigeon pose

Another famous stretch in yoga, Pigeon pose gives the hips a deep stretch. This pose is tough to perform, so people need to use caution when trying it for the first time.

To carryout this stretch:

    a. Start out in higher plank, as although doing a push-up.
    b. Lift the left foot and convey the knee directly forward toward the left hand, and push the foot towards the proper hand.
    c. Move the outstretched proper leg as a ways again as possible.
    d. Keeping the hips straight, decrease the physique to the ground as a long way as possible.

e. After a few seconds, swap sides.

CHAPTER FIVE

HIP FLEXOR STRENGTHENING EXERCISES YOU SHOULD PERFORM

Many hip flexor strengthening exercises can be carried out at the gym, even though they can also be performed at home.

There are some true workouts that can be done at home or the gym.

These exercises make stronger the legs in ordinary but goal the muscle groups that make up the hip flexors.

To fortify the hip flexor a man or woman can try the following:

Mountain climbers

Mountain climbers are certain moves a person does from a plank-like posture. Mountain climbers mimic the motion of mountain climbing up rocks, which is the place the title comes from.

To carryout mountain climbers:

a. Start in a normal plank with hands and toes placed shoulder-width apart.
b. Keep the palms firmly planted on the floor and pull the proper knee up to

the chest on the same side of the body.

c. Then, return to the starting role and repeat with the left leg.

Start off with 5 to 10 repetitions and build up to about 20 to 30 over time.

Lunges

Lunges are an incredible exercise to toughen the leg and hip muscles. People can operate lunges in a variety of ways, consisting of forward, backward, and toward either side. The simplest is a forward lunge.

To carryout a forward lunge:

    a. Start in a standing role with feet just slightly apart.
    b. Place palms on the hips or let them dangle straight on either aspect of the body.
    c. Take a huge step forward, making sure the heel makes contact with the ground first.
    d. Bend the forward knee till the thigh is parallel to the ground and

the knee is over the ankle while bending the different knee in the direction of the ground.
e. Step returned into the stand position, pushing off the flooring with the leading foot.
Repeat, alternating sides.

To start, 5 to 10 repetitions might also be all that a man or woman can do. However, constructing up to 20 to 30 repetitions is a true number to goal for.

Straight leg raises

Straight leg raises are any other exercising that can be executed lying down and involves lifting one leg at a time. It is easy to operate but gives the lower body a suitable workout.

To carryout the straight leg raise:

a. Start off lying on the floor with arms to the side.
b. Keeping feet on the floor, carry them towards the buttocks, forming a triangle with the knees.
c. Alternate lifting one leg then the other, developing a straight line from the hips to the ankle.
d. Repeat eight to 10 instances per leg.

Percy T. Williams

Squats

Squats are an extremely good way to reinforce hip muscles.

Squats can work the muscle tissues of the legs and engage the core at the equal time. Squats have an delivered benefit of being very flexible, that means a person can adjust the depth to in shape their changing health needs.

To carryout a squat:

 a. Start in a standing function with ft barely spread aside and palms to the side.
 b. Bend the knees and push the buttocks towards the back.
 c. Drop down till the legs are roughly parallel to the floor, keeping knees in line with the feet.
 d. Keep the abs tight and convey the fingers up to chest level.

e. Repeat 10 to 30 instances depending on fitness level.

As strength grows, human beings can add can jumps or weights for an extra challenge.

Clamming

Clamming is a popular exercise amongst dancers, who need to have robust hip muscle tissue to help with rotation. Initially, human beings can do clamming except resistance.

To operate a clam, a character should:

    a. Lay on their side with legs stacked on pinnacle of every different and slightly bent at the knee.
    b. Open the pinnacle knee so that it factors at the ceiling.
    c. While opening the knee, hold the feet stacked collectively and do now not roll backward on the bottom hip.
    d. To end the rep, close the leg.
    e. Repeat 10 to 30 instances per side.

People who have been doing this workout for a whilst can also use a therapy band for introduced resistance.

Hip abduction machines

People who have get admission to to a gymnasium may additionally be able to locate machines geared toward strengthening the hip flexors. Often seated, these machines focal point on squeezing the legs together or pushing them apart.

If focusing on the legs, a character should no longer pass by these machines at the gym, as they can help to improve the hip flexors.

CHAPTER SIX

RISKS ASSOCIATED WITH TIGHT HIP FLEXORS

Tight hip flexors can cause some practicable problems in unique parts of the body. Tight hip flexors can do the following:

1. Limit mobility
2. Cause lower lower back pain
3. Lead to on foot abnormally
4. Reduce speed
5. Cause pain in the hips
6. Increase the chance of harm when exercising
7. Lead to long-term hip trouble

CHAPTER SEVEN

WHAT DIFFERENT TREATMENT APPROACH IS AVALIABLE?

For minor hip flexor injuries, people do no longer typically visit their health practitioner however decides on to deal with themselves from home.

Some common approaches to help deal with hip flexor strain are:

a. Resting the muscular tissues to assist them to heal while heading off things to do that should cause further strain.

b. Wearing a compression wrap round the area. These are accessible to buy in pharmacies or online.
c. Applying an ice pack to the affected area. These are accessible to buy in pharmacies or online.
d. Applying a warmth pack to the affected area. These are on hand to purchase in pharmacies or online.
e. A hot bathe or bath.
f. Over-the-counter pain relievers, such as ibuprofen (Advil, Motrin), acetaminophen (Tylenol), naproxen sodium (Aleve).

When taking these medicines, it is necessary to follow the directions and not to use them for greater than 10 days.

If the pain persists after 10 days, a man or woman may additionally want to make an appointment with their doctor to discuss alternative treatments.

Surgery

In more severe cases, a doctor will generally advise an X-ray, MRI, or CT scan to confirm whether or not the bone has been fractured.

When the injury is strangely extensive, a medical doctor may additionally propose that an character sees a bodily therapist or undergoes surgical treatment to restore the muscle. However, cases of damage this severe are rare.

If hip flexor stress motives a limp or the signs and symptoms do no longer get higher after resting and treating at domestic for a week, it can also be really useful to see a doctor.

CHAPTER EIGHT

IMPORTANT TIPS TO PREVENT HIP FLEXOR

People who are especially vulnerable to hip flexor strain, such as athletes or these who generally participate in vigorous activities that should injury or overstretch the hip flexors, can take precautions to avoid injury.

Ensuring muscular tissues are true warmed up before taking section in physical activity, and doing exercises to reinforce the muscles, can assist to maintain the vicinity bendy and strong, and minimize the chances of injury happening.

THE END

Percy T. Williams

Tight Hip Flexor

Percy T. Williams

Tight Hip Flexor

www.ingramcontent.com/pod-product-compliance
Lightning Source LLC
Chambersburg PA
CBHW030544220526
45463CB00007B/2970